The Future of Antidepressants

The New Wave of Research

ANTIDEPRESSANTS

ANTIDEPRESSANTS:

The Future of Antidepressants

The New Wave of Research

by Heather Docalavich

Mason Crest Publishers

Philadelphia

Mason Crest Publishers Inc.
370 Reed Road
Broomall, Pennsylvania 19008
(866) MCP-BOOK (toll free)

First printing
1 2 3 4 5 6 7 8 9 10
Library of Congress Cataloging-in-Publication Data

Docalavich, Heather.
   The future of antidepressants : the new wave of research / by
Heather Docalavich.
      p. cm. — (Antidepressants)
   Includes bibliographical references and index.
   ISBN 1-4222-0103-1   ISBN 1-4222-0094-9 (series)
   1. Antidepressants—Juvenile literature.   I. Title. II. Series.
RM332.D62 2007
615'.78—dc22
                                                    2006010764

Interior design by MK Bassett-Harvey.
Interiors produced by Harding House Publishing Service, Inc.
www.hardinghousepages.com.
Cover design by Peter Culatta.
Printed in the Hashemite Kingdom of Jordan.

Contents

Introduction

by Andrew M. Kleiman, M.D.

From ancient Greece through the twenty-first century, the experience of sadness and depression is one of the many that define humanity. As long as human beings have felt emotions, they have endured depression. Experienced by people from every race, socioeconomic class, age group, and culture, depression is an emotional and physical experience that millions of people suffer each day. Despite being described in literature and music; examined by countless scientists, philosophers, and thinkers; and studied and treated for centuries, depression continues to remain as complex and mysterious as ever.

In today's Western culture, hearing about depression and treatments for depression is common. Adolescents in particular are bombarded with information, warnings, recommendations, and suggestions. It is critical that adolescents and young people have an understanding of depression and its impact on an individual's psychological and physical health, as well as the treatment options available to help those who suffer from depression.

Why? Because depression can lead to poor school performance, isolation from family and friends, alcohol and drug abuse, and even suicide. This doesn't have to be the case, since many useful and promising treatments exist to relieve the suffering of those with depression. Treatments for depression may also pose certain risks, however.

Since the beginning of civilization, people have been trying to alleviate the suffering of those with depression. Modern-day medicine and psychology have taken the understanding and treatment of depression to new heights. Despite their shortcomings, these treatments have helped millions and millions of people lead happier, more fulfilling and prosperous lives that would not be possible in generations past. These treatments, however, have their own risks, and for some people, may not be effective at all. Much work in neuroscience, medicine, and psychology needs to be done in the years to come.

Many adolescents experience depression, and this book series will help young people to recognize depression both in themselves and in those around them. It will give them the basic understanding of the history of depression and the various treatments that have been used to combat depression over the years. The books will also provide a basic scientific understanding of depression, and the many biological, psychological, and alternative treatments available to someone suffering from depression today.

Each person's brain and biology, life experiences, thoughts, and day-to-day situations are unique. Similarly, each individual experiences depression and sadness in a unique way. Each adolescent suffering from depression thus requires a distinct, individual treatment plan that best suits his or her needs. This series promises to be a vital resource for helping young people recognize and understand depression, and make informed and thoughtful decisions regarding treatment.

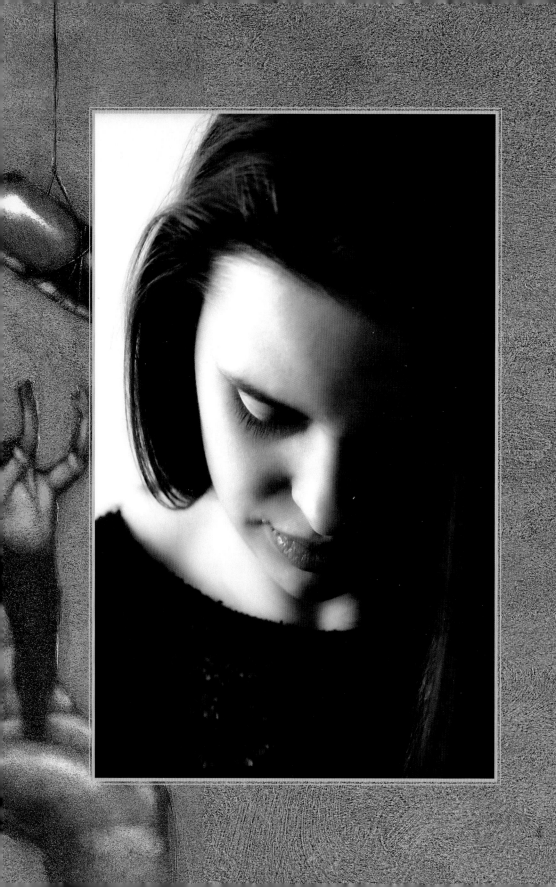

Chapter 1

Evolving Theories on the Causes of Depression

David wanted to know why his mom was the way she was. Even in his earliest memories she had always seemed out of sync with everyone else. One day she could be normal, and later she would be "down" even when they were supposed to be having a good time, like at his birthday parties or trips to the zoo.

David knew that was why his dad had left the family. His father had been gone for years now. David was angry with his father for leaving his mother on her own when she was so unable to cope, but at the same time he wondered if anyone could ever really be happy with his mom.

David's mother had been diagnosed years ago with ***clinical depression***. Even when his mom was on her "meds" she was difficult; besides, she said she hated the side effects and she never felt well. When she was off her medication, David often had to go stay with his grandmother.

David's grandmother talked about the regrets she had about her daughter's childhood. Apparently, his mom hadn't grown up in a very happy home either. David and his grandmother spent many Friday nights in her tiny kitchen wondering out loud whether it had been the death of David's grandfather when his mother was still a young girl that had sent her into depression—or if it was an inherited problem. One of

What Is Depression?

Depression is the most common major mood disorder and involves changes in a person's emotions, behavior, and thought patterns, changes that are strong enough to disrupt a person's usual functioning for six months or more. Although depression may seem like a temporary "down-in-the-dumps" mood, the sufferer cannot simply "cheer up" after a while. Everyone gets sad now and then, but unlike a usual "blue" mood, the symptoms of depression may last for weeks, months, or even, in some cases, years. A person with depression typically experiences depressive episodes, periods during which she is depressed, several times over the course of her life.

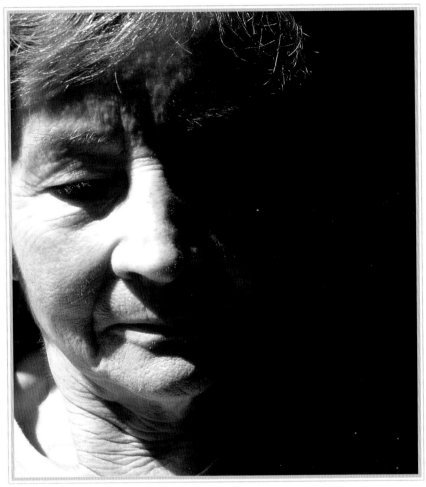

Depression sometimes runs in families.

his mother's paternal aunts had also been depressed and had once attempted suicide.

It frustrated both David and his grandmother that the doctors could never tell them why this had happened to their family. David also harbored a secret fear: what if he inherited

What Are the Symptoms of Depression?

• *feelings of extreme sadness, emptiness, anxiety*

• *thoughts of hopelessness, helplessness*

• *thoughts of suicide, suicide attempts*

• *loss of interest in usual activities, such as hobbies, school, or work*

• *loss of appetite or overeating*

• *oversleeping or waking up unusually early, and difficulty sleeping*

• *loss of concentration, difficulty remembering*

• *fatigue*

• *restlessness or irritability*

• *physical symptoms such as headaches, backaches, and digestive trouble that do not improve with medical treatment*

Not everyone who is depressed suffers all of these symptoms; according to the Diagnostic and Statistical Manual for Mental Disorders, Fourth Edition (DSM-IV), a person must suffer from at least five of the above symptoms to be considered to be having a major depressive episode.

this disease from his mother? He wished the doctors would hurry and find the cause of his mother's illness; maybe then they could make sure she got better. As things were, he sometimes wondered if the doctors knew all that much more than he did about what had caused his mother's depression.

Suspected Biological Causes of Depression

The biological causes of clinical depression are perhaps studied more extensively than any other theories of depression's origins. Over the last few decades much progress has been made in understanding brain function, the roles of **neurotransmitters** and **hormones**, and other biological processes, as well as how they may relate to the development of mental illnesses like depression.

The brain controls all the basic functions of our bodies, our movements, and our thoughts and emotions. Scientists studying clinical depression have been researching several aspects of brain function, including the structures of the **limbic system** (a pattern of connections in the brain that is thought to control and regulate emotions) and the function of neurotransmitters and **neurons**.

Chemical Imbalance

Although the idea of a "chemical imbalance" has taken much of the blame for causing depression in the popular media, it is still unknown whether changes in levels of neurotransmitters actually cause the onset of depression—or if depression causes changes in neurotransmitters. It may work both ways. Some scientists also believe that our behavior can affect our brain chemistry, while others believe that brain chemistry causes certain behavior. For instance, if a person experiences a severe or ongoing trauma, this may cause her brain chemistry to be affected, leading to clinical depression. On the other hand, that same person may develop strategies to consciously change depressed thoughts and behavior and better deal with stressful events. Learning to do this can also change brain chemistry and may relieve depression.

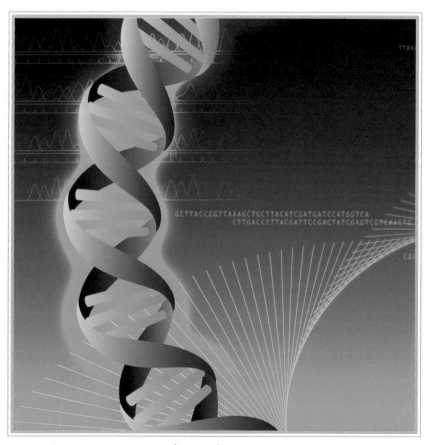

The DNA we inherit from our parents may make us more vulnerable to depression.

Clearly, the answer is not simple—but in a way, that's only to be expected. Although we often speak of emotions, behaviors, and physical ailments as three quite separate things, in reality, we cannot divide a human being into neat packages. Our bodies, minds, and emotions all interact with one another; they are seamless parts of a single whole.

The Endocrine System

Another area of study in finding the biological causes of clinical depression is focused on the endocrine system. The endocrine system, which works with the brain to control several different activities within the body, is made up of small glands that create hormones and release them into the bloodstream. These hormones regulate important processes such as reaction to stress and sexual development.

Scientists have found that many people who are depressed have abnormal levels of certain hormones in their blood despite having healthy glands. Researchers believe that such hormonal imbalances are related to some of depression's symptoms—such as problems with appetite and sleep—since hormones normally help regulate these activities.

The Role of Genetics

Doctors have known for many years that depressive illnesses can run in families. Researchers who study depression have been able to show that to some degree, depressive illnesses can be inherited—but what individuals may actually inherit is not the disease itself but a ***vulnerability*** to depression. In other words, if a person has close family members who have clinical depression, he may inherit a tendency to develop the illness under certain circumstances. It does not necessarily mean, however, that he is automatically doomed to become depressed.

The genes that individuals inherit from their parents determine many things, such as height, whether a person is male or female, even eye and hair color. Every human cell contains somewhere between 50,000 and 100,000 genes. They are all made up of something called DNA, or deoxyribonucleic acid. Genes can be found on chromosomes within the nucleus of each cell. All of our cells, except sex cells, contain forty-six chromosomes, and each gene can usually be found in a specific place on a particular chromosome. No two people in the world have the exact same genetic makeup, except for identical twins.

Research on depression within families shows that certain people are more likely to develop the illness than others. If you have a parent or sibling who has had major depression, you may be three times more likely to develop the condition than those who do not have a close relative with the illness. You also have a much higher chance of developing **bipolar disorder**, another type of mood disorder. Since close relatives of people with clinical depression have such a susceptibility to developing the condition themselves, many scientists feel strongly that the disease has a genetic component.

Bipolar disorder has an even stronger genetic link. Of people with bipolar disorder, approximately half of them have a parent with some history of mood disorder. If a mother or father has bipolar disorder, their child has a one in four chance of developing some type of mood disorder. When both parents have bipolar disorder, the chance of their child also developing bipolar disorder rises to between 50 and 75 percent. Siblings of individuals with bipolar disorder may be up to eighteen times more likely to develop bipolar disorder, and up to ten times more likely to develop major depressive disorder than others with no such brothers or sisters. Clearly, genetics plays a role in the development of mood disorders, including depression and bipolar disorder.

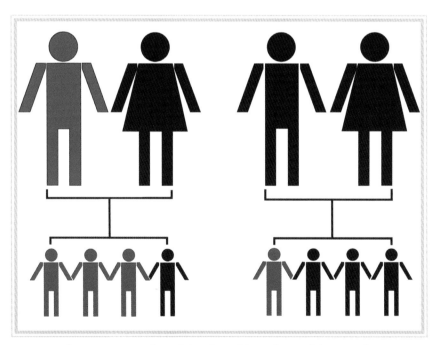

If one parent has bipolar disorder, odds are that one out four of their children will also have this disorder. If both parents have bipolar disorder, as many as three out of four of their children may develop this disorder at some point in their lives.

How Environmental Causes May Influence Depression

People have long understood that environment can affect state of mind. Our relationships, our childhoods, losses we

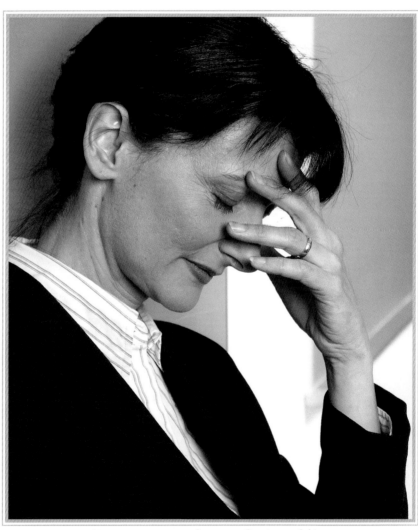

Stress in our personal or professional lives may contribute to the onset of depression.

suffer, and the stress we face all affect our thoughts, emotions, and behaviors. How we react to these circumstances in our environment may influence the development of clinical depression.

There appears to be some relationship between stressful situations, our reaction to stress, and the onset of depressive illness. Many people develop depression after a stressful event in their lives. Events like the death of a loved one, the loss of a job, or a divorce are often difficult and cause great pain for many people. But stress can also occur as the result of a positive event, such as getting married, moving, or changing jobs.

Researchers don't yet fully understand whether a stressful event itself can actually cause a person to become depressed. All of us struggle with hardships at different points in our lives. Most of the time, these difficult situations do not directly cause depression. On the other hand, some people become depressed even when there is little or no visible stress in their lives and things seem to be going fine. No one single event predictably causes depression to develop in every person. While one type of stressor may lead to depression in one person, it may cause only a passing blue mood for another.

Research shows that if a stressful experience causes a person to become depressed, it probably works indirectly. For example, if a young man with a family history of major depression suffers the loss of a high-paying job, he may become clinically depressed. It is not necessarily the loss of the job itself that caused the development of depression, but a genetic predisposition combined with the stressful event that made him more vulnerable.

For people with **chronic** depression, the emotional effects of environment may be more complicated. A stressful event such as a job loss or the death of a loved one is likely to come before a first or second depressive episode. After that, future depressive episodes can develop **spontaneously**, without a stressor preceding the episode. No one is sure why stress seems to lead to depression in this way. However, researchers

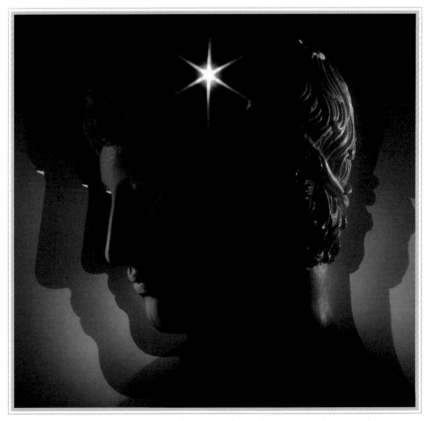

A depressive episode may be like a spark inside a person's brain chemistry, kindling a blazing fire.

have developed an explanation called the "kindling effect," or "kindling-sensitization hypothesis."

This theory assumes that the first depressive episodes spark changes in the brain's chemistry and limbic system that make the person more prone to developing further episodes of depression. Just as small sparks from kindling help to build a blazing fire, early episodes of depression make a person more sensitive, so that even small environmental stressors can lead to later depressive episodes.

While some depression stems from a single traumatic event, other people may become depressed as a result of having to live with chronic stress. Such stress may come in the form of having to juggle multiple roles at home and work, making changes in one's lifestyle, or being in an abusive environment. They may also come with everyday life changes, such as late adolescence and early adulthood when many people separate from their families to establish their own independence. Likewise, middle age can require adjustment to changes in sexuality, children leaving the home, and concerns about employment. Retirement is another time of major life changes when some people struggle with health problems and finances. When a person is under these sorts of constant stress, a single difficult event is much more likely to cause a depressive episode. In other words, an initial depressive episode may "prime" the brain for further episodes.

Imagine a middle-aged woman in an unhappy marriage: she may be more likely to become depressed after her youngest child leaves home for college. The event of her child leaving home may not by itself have been enough to cause depression, but the constant stress of marital problems combined with this event may be significant enough to trigger clinical depression.

Depressed people have also generally experienced more difficulties in childhood than those who do not become depressed. The most significant event that seems to be related to clinical depression is separation from or death of a parent before the age of eleven. Abuse (sexual, physical, and emotional), neglect, and an unstable home environment can also create problems for children when they reach adulthood.

While scientists do not completely understand how childhood traumas can result in adult depression, they have a few theories. One theory suggests that children who experience great sadness growing up have a harder time adjusting to later changes in their life, such as puberty and the increased responsibilities of adulthood. Another theory is that these children may not attain appropriate emotional maturity or they become otherwise emotionally damaged, which in turn, makes them vulnerable to depression. Still another theory on how environment influences depression has to do with the developing brain of a young child. An infant's earliest experiences may affect the development of the limbic system in the brain. Scientists theorize that when an infant experiences great emotional distress, this could affect her ability later in life to adapt to new environments and regulate emotions.

While many different theories on the causes of clinical depression have been put forth, no definitive answer has yet been found. At present, the best information points toward a combination of genetic and environmental factors influencing the depressed patient's biology. New research is helping us to have a far greater understanding of the biology of depression and to build a new arsenal of antidepressant drugs to combat this destructive illness.

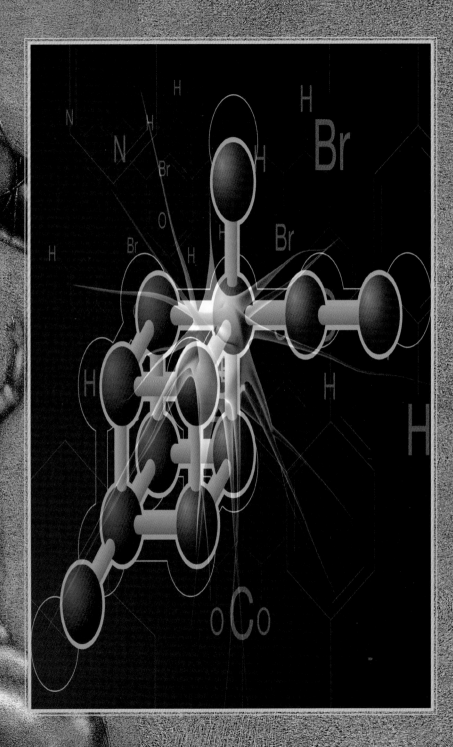

Chapter 2

From Chemical Imbalance to Nerve-Cell Connections

Leslie is waiting in her mom's car for the examiner to get in on the passenger side. Although she is very excited to take her road test again, she's nervous too. Really nervous, almost like she might get sick. Her heart is pounding in her chest, her hands are sweaty and slick on the steering wheel, and on top of her queasy stomach, her whole body is suffering from a feeling of general shakiness. It seems like she has never been so aware of the minute hand on her watch. The examiner should be here any minute. Hopefully she won't fail her driver's test this time.

While Leslie is very aware of her surroundings, of the time, and of being stressed out over her road test, thousands of things are happening inside Leslie's body, things she has no clue are happening. For example, her brain is busy interpreting Leslie's fear and anxiety and sending messages out to her body to prepare it for upcoming trauma. Leslie's brain has no way to tell the difference between the stress of an upcoming road test and the kind of stress faced by our early human ancestors, who might have been facing down a much more serious threat, like a predator. Her brain, prepared to react this

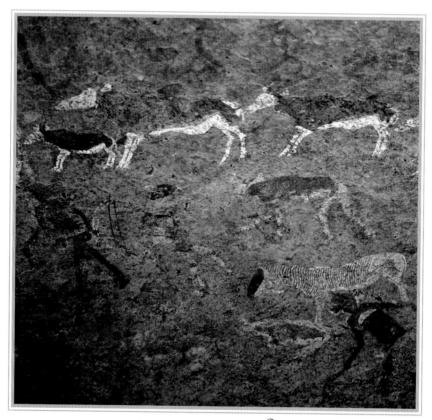

Our ancestors' brains were designed to deal with the concrete dangers of hunting food; in the modern world, we face different sources of stress.

way over thousands of years, is busy sending out messages to cells all over Leslie's body.

Messages move from one nerve cell to another in Leslie's brain, first as electrical impulses, later converted into chemical messages. In Leslie's current situation, the messages being transmitted are designed to increase her heart rate and respiration in case she suddenly needs to flee from the scene of her road test; the brain transmits all its messages the same way. So at the moment Leslie's brain is sending the necessary signals to prepare her to face danger, it is also regulating her breathing and heartbeat, telling her muscles how to move to drive the car; interpreting the input from her senses so that she can feel, see, and hear; and all the while regulating her mood. Although Leslie is completely unaware of all this activity, the chemistry and healthy functioning of her brain is impacting every aspect of her life.

Understanding the Chemical Imbalance

For years people have believed clinical depression to be simply the result of a chemical imbalance in the brain. According to this theory, a person has too little of one or another critical compound and brain chemistry is thrown out of whack, causing a depressive illness. The theory of the chemical imbalance originated when the first antidepressant medications were discovered. These drugs boosted the level of certain brain chemicals, and for many patients, their depression lifted. Problem solved. Or at least so it seemed, until scientists realized that the new drugs, while effective for many, didn't help everybody. Today we realize that the biological causes of depression are likely to be far more complicated.

Special chemicals called neurotransmitters carry out many very important tasks within the brain. Their main job is to help transfer messages between the brain's nerve cells. These nerve cells, called neurons, are each designed to control specific activities. We have anywhere from ten billion to one hundred billion neurons within our brains. Anytime we react in any way, feel, or think, our neurons send messages in the form of electrical impulses from one cell to another.

A neuron is made up of smaller parts: a cell body, an axon, and numerous branches called dendrites. Messages are passed through the brain by traveling through these special structures. First, one of the branches or dendrites of the neuron pick up an electrical impulse. From there, the impulse moves through the cell body and then travels down the axon. When the impulse reaches the axon, it is transformed from an electrical impulse to a chemical impulse. These chemicals, or neurotransmitters, are then released by the axon with the task of carrying the messages from this neuron to the next. When the message is picked up by the dendrite of a neighboring neuron, it is changed back into an electrical impulse and the whole process starts over. Neurons never actually touch each other. Instead, the neurotransmitters pass from one neuron to the next through a narrow channel, called a synapse, which separates the neurons.

Neurotransmitters operate in a very orderly and structured way. Their molecules are specially shaped so that after they leave a neuron and pass into the synapse, they can be received at precise sites, called receptors, on a neighboring neuron. When the chemical message lands at the neuron's receptor site, the neurotransmitter may either be changed into an electrical impulse and continue on its way through the next neuron, or it may stay where it is. Whatever happens, the neurotransmitter is eventually released from the receptor site and flows back into the synapse. It finally leaves the synapse in one of two ways. Sometimes neurotransmitters may be broken down. At other times, they may reconnect to a receptor site on the neuron that originally released them, in a process called reuptake.

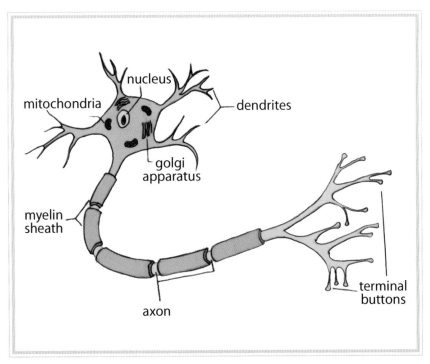

A nerve cell

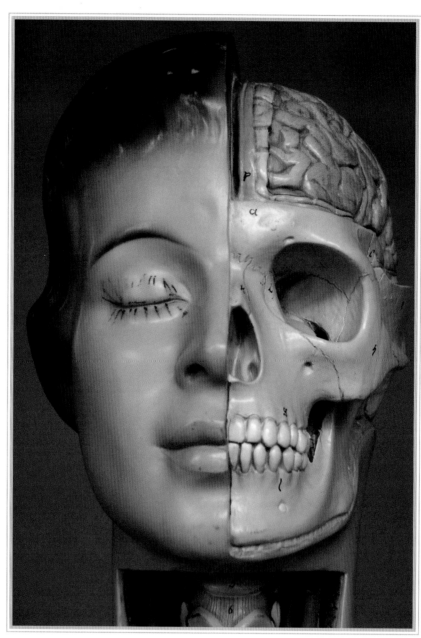

Researchers cannot simply peel back a person's skin and bone and look inside the brain, the way they might be able to do with another body organ; scientists still don't understand exactly how the brain functions.

So far, scientists have identified about thirty different neu-rotransmitters. Researchers have discovered a link between clinical depression and the function of three neurotransmit-ters: serotonin, norepinephrine, and dopamine. These three neurotransmitters are found in parts of the brain that regu-late our emotions, reactions to stress, and the physical drives of sleep, appetite, and sexuality.

Original theories about how neurotransmitters may be re-lated to a person's mood were based on the effects that antide-pressant medications were observed to have on patients. The earliest antidepressant drugs were discovered almost by coin-cidence, and later, doctors tried to discover *why* they worked. Scientists now believe these medications are effective because they regulate the amount of specific neurotransmitters in the brain. However, the role that neurotransmitters play in the development or treatment of clinical depression is still not completely clear.

For instance, many people who are depressed have low lev-els of the neurotransmitter norepinephrine. This is a simple example that seems to validate the "chemical imbalance" the-ory of how depression occurs. If someone with depression has a low level of norepinephrine, the use of some antidepressants can increase the level of norepinephrine in the brain, and should then relieve the person's symptoms. Unfortunately, the problem is not nearly so simple. For one thing, research-ers have found that some other people who are depressed have very *high* levels of norepinephrine. Because there are so many different kinds of neurotransmitters, including perhaps some that have not yet been discovered, researchers cannot point to one or two chemicals as the culprits responsible for causing depression. What's more, antidepressant medications do not work for everyone.

If the level of a neurotransmitter in the brain was directly linked to depression, then we would expect a much higher rate of success with medication. To make things still more confusing, antidepressant medications change the level of a neurotransmitter in the brain immediately, but a person with depression normally needs to be on an antidepressant for a few weeks to feel better. Ultimately, while scientists have found a strong relationship between neurotransmitter levels in the brain and clinical depression—and antidepressant medications certainly work for a great many people—we are still uncertain of the actual relationship between neurotransmitters and depressive illness. It may be that there are many different types or sub-types of depression with different biological mechanisms and various transmitters playing a role.

Understanding Nerve-Cell Connections

Scientists are continuously making new discoveries about the biology of depression, with the goal of developing better treatments. According to the new research, depression may stem not from a chemical imbalance but from unhealthy nerve-cell connections in the areas of the brain that create our emotions. If that's true—and the evidence to support that theory is growing stronger—then the real goal of medicine is not to change the brain's chemistry but to repair its faulty circuitry.

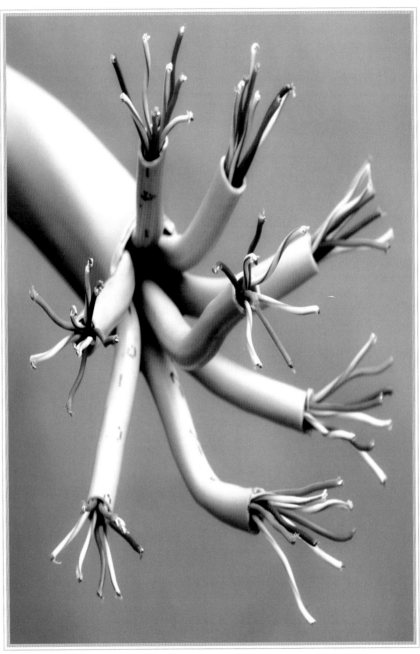

If you think of the body's messages as electricity, then a breakdown in the electrical wires (connections between nerve cells) may explain depression.

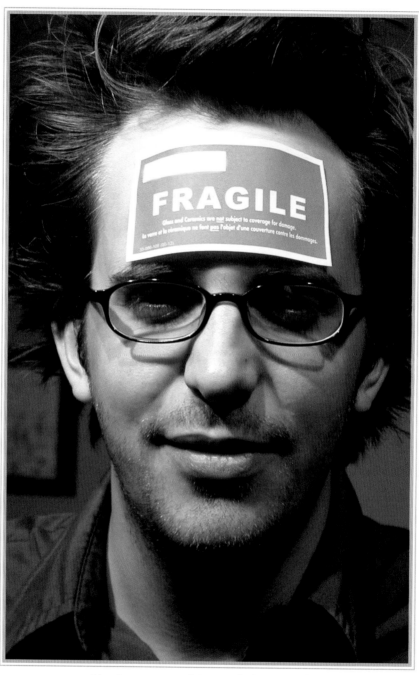

*The inner workings of the mind are
complicated and fragile.*

Scientists researching clinical depression have been focusing on a particular part of the brain called the limbic system. This is the part of the brain that controls activities like our emotions, physical and sexual drives, and the stress response. Various areas of the limbic system have special importance. The hypothalamus, for example, is a small structure located at the base of the brain that regulates many basic functions such as body temperature, sleep, appetite, sex drive, stress reaction, and other body activities. The hypothalamus also controls the function of the pituitary gland, which in turn controls our hormones. Other structures within the limbic system that are associated with our emotions and mood are the ***amygdala*** and hippocampus. The activities of the limbic system are so complex that trouble in any part of it, including how neurotransmitters function, could affect mood or behavior.

The new frontiers of research reflect a growing awareness of how chronic distress affects the brain. Our stress-hormone system, which is designed to boost us into a state of extreme awareness and anxiety in an emergency, may remain "switched on" in susceptible people, especially those who were traumatized in childhood. Overexposure to stress hormones slows the growth of nerve cells in an area of the brain called the hippocampus. This brain center allows us to take in sensory input, link our experiences to our emotions, and store the combined information as our memories. The hippocampus is usually smaller in depressed people, with many brain cells lost and some shrunken. Experts suspect unlocking the secrets of the hippocampus will be critical to the further understanding of depression.

The theory that depression is linked to delayed nerve-cell growth or damaged connections may explain an old mystery. Since antidepressant medications boost neurotransmitter levels immediately, why does it often take six weeks or more to feel better? Recent studies show us that antidepressants stimulate the growth of new hippocampal nerve cells, which form new connections with older nerve cells. This process takes several weeks.

New Treatments Based on These Theories

If antidepressant drugs like Prozac® ease depression by inadvertently boosting the creation of new nerve cells, then scientists believe that drugs designed specifically for that purpose might bring faster and improved relief while causing fewer side effects. Researchers are already pursuing several possible options.

One strategy is to find a drug to hinder the action of Substance P, one of the chemical messengers involved in stress response. Unfortunately, aprepitant, the first Substance P blocker to be put into clinical trials, has recently proved worthless as an antidepressant. (Clinical trials are discussed more in chapter 4.) However, more similar compounds are still under study, and researchers are hoping to develop a Substance P blocker that will work.

A second possible compound for study is corticotrophin-releasing hormone (CRH), a chemical produced by the hypothalamus, a tiny structure of the brain with the huge responsibility of integrating hormones with behavior. CRH starts a

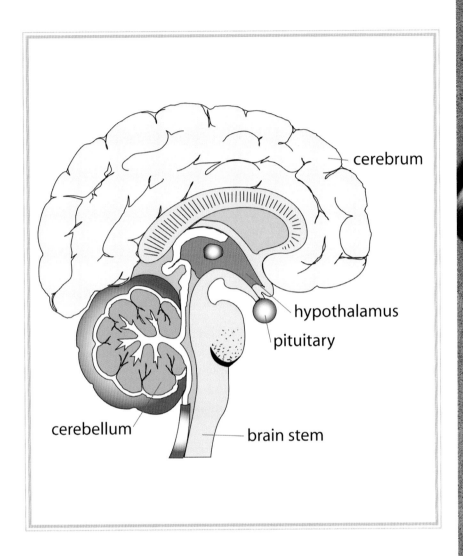

reaction that results in the release of the stress hormone cortisol into the bloodstream. Researchers have recently shown that an experimental CRH blocker called R121919 can slow down the stress response both in lab animals and in depressed patients. While that drug was eventually abandoned due to concerns about liver damage, drug companies are now developing other CRH blockers and working to understand other parts of the stress response.

Drugs that suppress vasopressin, another hormone released under conditions of stress, leave rats less anxious and more energetic in lab tests. Drugs that imitate a stress-reducing hormone called Neuropeptide Y also have similar effects. In lab tests, they also have the ability to decrease a mouse's need for alcohol, pointing the way to a promising new treatment for alcoholism. None of these drugs have reached advanced stages of clinical research, but some researchers believe they represent the future of antidepressants.

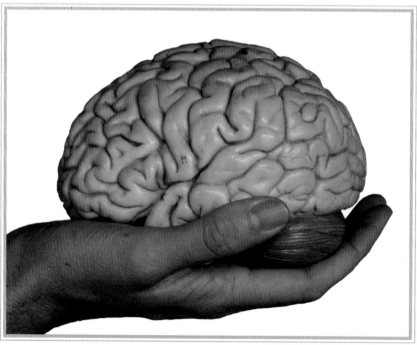

The brain may truly be the "final frontier," one of the last, uncharted regions for humanity to explore.

It may still take us decades to understand the complex biology of depression. The brain is truly a vast and uncharted territory that scientists are only beginning to map. In the meantime, a tremendous amount of government, private, and industry research money is going toward understanding and treating depression. For individuals confronting the reality of depression, new treatments that work offer the hope of a better life.

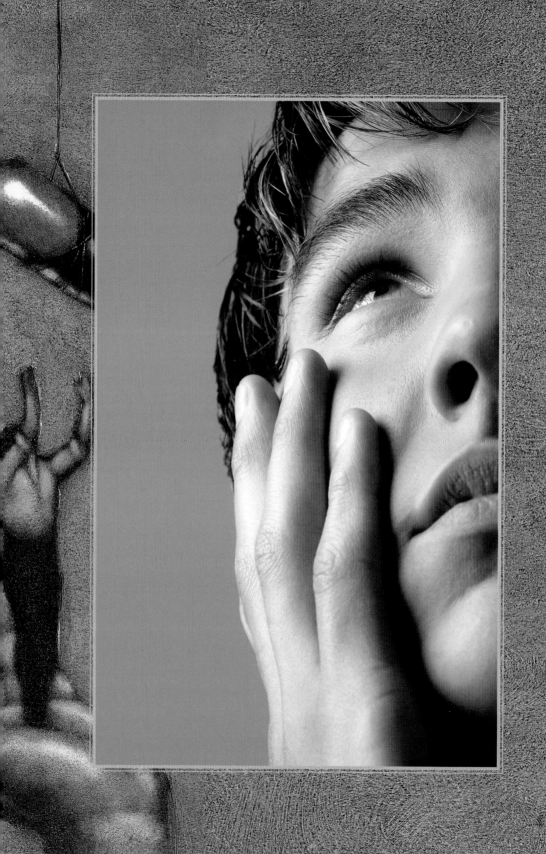

Chapter 3

It's All Hormones—
Or Is It All Stress?

Bill was walking on eggshells this week. He never knew how his girlfriend, Melissa, was going to react to anything these days. It just didn't seem like he could do anything right anymore. One minute she would seem like her normal, cheerful, outgoing self. The next, she was crying and depressed—or else she was angry and irritated by everything he said.

Bill and Melissa had been dating only a month, and at first, everything was great. However, the last week had been a nightmare. One night she even got mad at him in front of her mom and stormed out of the room. It had been pretty awkward standing there in the living room alone with Melissa's mom, but she had tried to smooth things over. "Don't worry, Bill," she said. "Melissa's always a little difficult around this time of the month."

Bill thought that was a pretty poor excuse for the way Melissa had been acting, but he didn't understand the changes that were going on inside her body, especially in her brain. As the hormones that regulate Melissa's reproductive system were shifting to prepare for menstruation, they were affecting the reactions of her body to many of the other hormones and chemicals that are critical to maintaining normal functioning. In Melissa's case, these reproductive hormones were probably causing her moods to fluctuate more rapidly and intensely than normal.

Bill's brain chemistry was changing too. His own reproductive hormones had little to do with it, since changes in men's sex hormones do not usually cause the mood swings found in some women. Instead, his brain was busy sending out messages to his glands to produce more of a hormone called cortisol, which helps us to cope with stressful situations. Bill was feeling the effects of this change as increased anxiety. Of course, neither he nor Melissa was aware of the complex chemical reactions that kept them mentally healthy from day to day.

How Hormones Can Affect Mood

Hormones are chemicals in the body that tell cells what to do. Hormonal changes may be connected to the changes in brain chemistry that are seen in people with clinical depression. As we mentioned earlier, the endocrine system is connected to the brain by the hypothalamus, which controls many important body functions, such as sleep, appetite, and sexual drive. The hypothalamus also controls the pituitary gland that, in turn, regulates hormone levels. The hypothalamus uses the neurotransmitters that are linked to depression—such as serotonin, norepinephrine, and dopamine—to manage hormone function. Sometimes, depression may be a symptom of a disease that affects the organs that produce our hormones. Examples of these types of diseases include thyroid disorders, Cushing's syndrome, and Addison's disease.

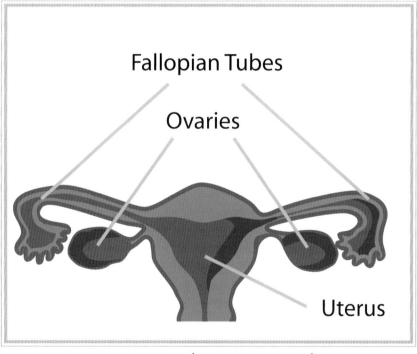

Fallopian Tubes

Ovaries

Uterus

A woman's reproductive system releases hormones that affect her emotions.

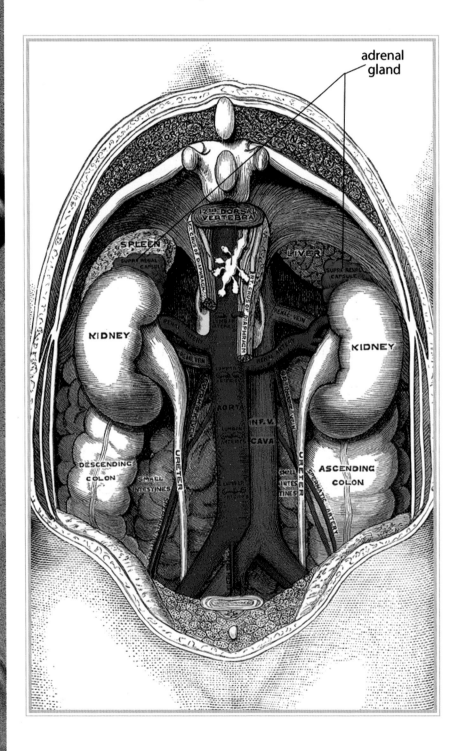

adrenal
gland

Cortisol

Of people who are clinically depressed, about half will have an excess of the hormone cortisol. Cortisol is a hormone made by the adrenal glands. Located near the kidneys, the adrenal glands help us to react to stress. Cortisol can continue to be produced even when someone already has high levels in her blood. The high cortisol levels usually return to a normal level once the depression disappears.

Scientists think that the hypothalamus may be responsible for abnormally high levels of cortisol in the blood, since it starts the process that leads to the production of cortisol by the adrenal glands. The hypothalamus first makes CRH. The pituitary gland then releases adrenocorticotrophic hormone (ACTH), which tells the adrenal glands to release cortisol into the blood. When a person's endocrine system is healthy, the hypothalamus controls the level of cortisol that is in the blood. If the level rises, the hypothalamus slows down its influence on the pituitary gland in production of CRH. When cortisol levels become reduced, the hypothalamus causes the pituitary gland to produce more CRH. In a person who is depressed, the hypothalamus may continuously tell the pituitary to produce CRH regardless of the amount of cortisol that is in the blood.

Female Reproductive Hormones

Other hormones may also play an important role in depression. Women have a far higher lifetime risk for depression than men; in fact, twice as many women as men will develop depression. Although the rate of bipolar disorder in men and women is almost equal, the course of that illness may differ between the sexes. Men may be more prone to develop periods of *mania*, whereas women may be more likely to experience periods of depression. This has led researchers to ask: "What are the contributing factors to the higher rate of depression in women?"

It now seems likely that reproductive hormones play an important role in mood changes. Studies of *estrogen* treatment for mood disorders have shown that too much or too little estrogen can change a person's mood. For example, one study found that estrogen caused rapid mood cycles in *postmenopausal* women with depression, but when the estrogen was discontinued, the rapid mood cycles ceased. The *postpartum* period, a time where there is a rapid decline of reproductive hormone levels, is also a peak time for women to develop a mood disorder.

A stronger connection between the reproductive system and the thyroid may exist in women than in men. In women, levels of different reproductive hormones affect the release of the thyroid's hormones into the body. No similar effect has been seen in men. Women are also more likely to develop thyroid disorders, which can make them more vulnerable to rapid mood cycles. Fortunately, they are also more responsive to thyroid treatment. More research is necessary before scientists can fully understand the connection between reproductive hormones and mood disorders.

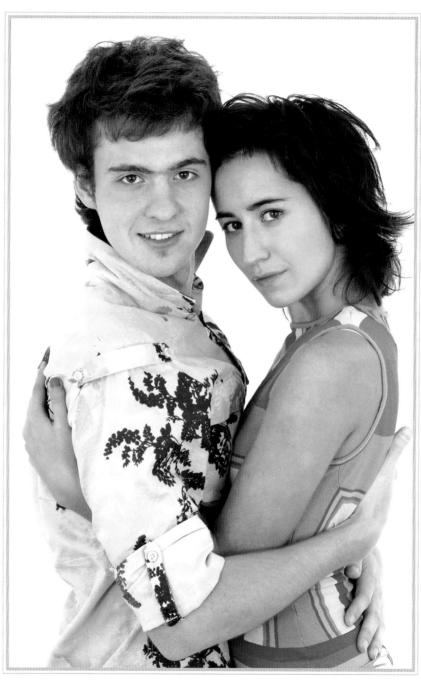

Because women and men have different hormone levels, women have different emotional experiences from men.

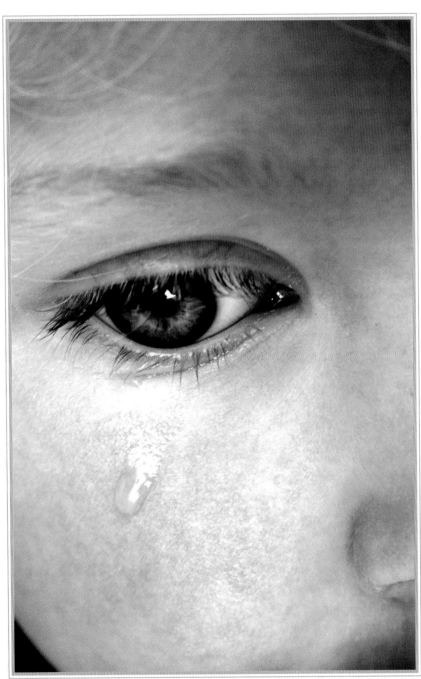

Childhood trauma, particularly sexual abuse, may make an individual more susceptible to depression as an adult.

The Role of Stress in Depression

Many researchers feel that abnormally high exposure to stress can cause hormonal changes to occur in the first place. Evidence from new research suggests that not only does trauma or stress suffered early in life or over an extended period of time play a role in developing depression, but brief or even one-time traumatic events can impact our brain chemistry.

In a study published in the August 2, 2000, *Journal of the American Medical Association*, forty-nine women were recruited for a depression study. The women were divided into four groups: those with no history of childhood abuse or psychiatric disorder, those with current major depression who had been physically or sexually abused as children, those without current major depression who had been physically or sexually abused as children, and those with current major depression with no history of childhood abuse. The women were then exposed to stressors such as math tests and being made to speak in public. Blood samples and heart readings showed that the women with a history of childhood abuse exhibited increased pituitary and ***autonomic responses*** (such as blood pressure, heart rate, and sweating) to the stress compared with the women who were not abused. This was especially true for the women with current depression and anxiety.

When a person is stressed, the hypothalamus in the brain secretes CRF, which results in the pituitary gland releasing another hormone, ACTH, which then activates the adrenal glands that turn loose the stress hormone cortisol. This neuroendocrine circuit is referred to as the HPA (hypotha-lamic-pituitary-adrenal) axis. The abused and depressed women in the study exhibited a sixfold greater ACTH increase over the control group. The women abused in childhood de-

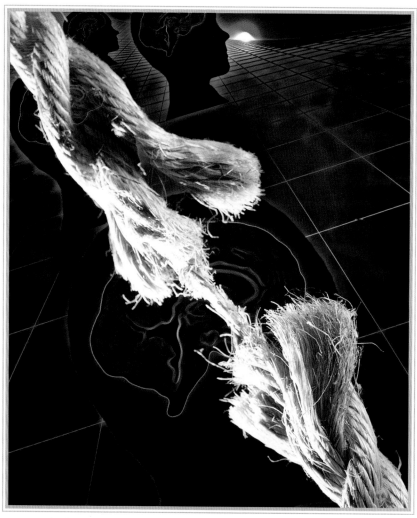

Each person's genetic background is unique, but when stress is combined with a genetic predisposition, an individual's probability of a major depression increases.

veloped a **sensitized** brain system, where CRF receptors were found in abundance. Depressed patients have extra high concentrations of CRF in their **cerebrospinal** fluid. Thus, childhood stress may predispose people to their hormones becoming disregulated, which in turn can lead to depression.

One-time occurrences such as divorce or death of a loved one also impact our mental health. A study of major depression in twins found that a recent stressful event was the single largest risk factor for an episode of major depression. According to the study, those with the lowest genetic risk of depression had only a 0.5 percent probability of depression that month, but this shot up to 6.2 percent with exposure to severe stress. Those with the highest genetic risk faced a 1.1 percent probability that skyrocketed to 14.6 percent when stress was present. In other words, stress plus a genetic predisposition often equals depression.

New Treatments Related to These Theories

The push to understand the connection between hormones, stress, and depression has led researchers to direct their attention to the chemicals involved in the control of our stress response system, as well as potential ways to interrupt that cycle in people where it appears to have gone awry.

As mentioned earlier, several studies have shown an overproduction of CRH in patients with depression and certain anxiety disorders. Newly discovered drugs called CRH blockers are designed to disrupt the action of these chemicals and represent a promising new kind of antidepressant. Such compounds can now be found in a wide range of preclinical studies for antidepressants and anxiety-relieving medications.

CRH blockers represent a exciting potential class of new medicines to treat anxiety and depression. Although R121919 is no longer being considered for clinical development, Bristol-Myers Squibb, Novartis, Pfizer, and Neurogen, and other large pharmaceutical companies are currently studying similar new compounds that are in various stages of preclinical and clinical development. While it is clear that additional research needs to be conducted, CRH blockers show promise as a new approach to treating depression.

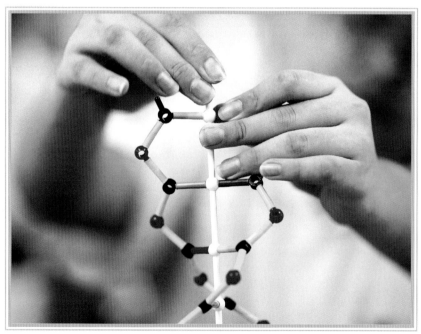

Researchers are seeking a way to create a protective gene that could increase serotonin production in the brain.

Another possible approach is the treatment of depression with beta-blockers, a class of medications used for reducing high blood pressure that have also been found to hamper the formation of emotionally disturbing memories. Beta-blockers occupy some adrenaline receptors, preventing adrenaline from transmitting information. Researchers hope to be able to harness the ability of beta-blockers to interfere with the stress response system as a means of alleviating depression.

Another potential treatment is gene therapy. Although the study of this potential treatment is currently in the earliest stages of development, the theory behind it is promising. In one ambitious study, scientists constructed a type of herpes virus responsive to cortisol and introduced it into the hippocampus of lab animals. The researchers' aim was to alter normal brain function during stress so that a protective gene can be switched on, say one that increases serotonin production.

The process of creating new antidepressants is often slow, since it usually requires years of research. Once a promising chemical has been developed, government agencies in the United States and Canada require that certain procedures be followed before it can be released to the public as a medicine.

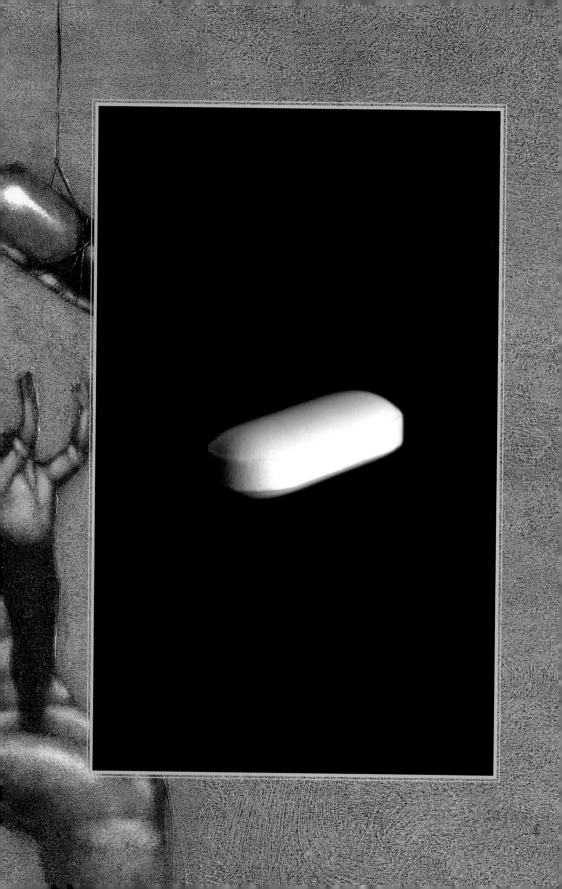

Chapter 4

Creating New Antidepressants

Every day Jeremy woke up and took his medicine with his breakfast. This tiny pill had really made a difference in his life. For more than a year he had suffered, not knowing exactly what the problem was but simply convinced that life no longer held the possibility of anything good for him. He stopped eating, he slept all day, he lost touch with his family and friends. The only constant in his life was the endless feeling of hopelessness.

Fortunately, Jeremy's best friend never gave up on him, and eventually, he convinced Jeremy to go to his doctor for help. The doctor had prescribed an antidepressant and referred Jeremy for counseling. At first, nothing changed, but over time, the dark fog that had taken over Jeremy's life had begun to lift. Now he felt better than he had at any time in

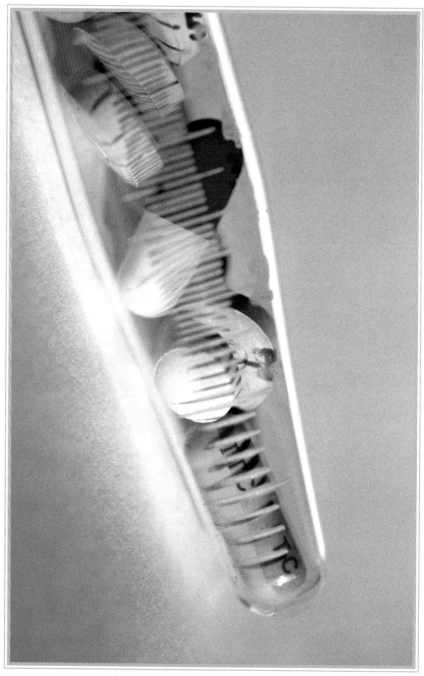

A medication is a substance that affects the body in a positive way.

recent memory, and he knew much of that was because of the tiny pill he took each day.

What Jeremy may never fully understand is the lengthy and complicated process that took an idea from the research laboratory and turned it into the medication in his hand.

What Is a Medication?

A medication is legally defined as "any substance (other than a food or device) intended for use in the diagnosis, cure, relief, treatment, or prevention of disease or intended to affect the structure or function of the body." This complex definition of a drug, although important for legal purposes, is rather complicated for everyday use. A simpler but useful definition of a medication is any chemical substance that affects the body and its processes.

The Government's Role

In the United States and Canada, strict laws control the production, sale, and use of drugs. Some drugs, like cocaine and marijuana, are illegal to sell, to use, or even to possess. The law also divides legal drugs into two categories: prescription drugs and nonprescription drugs. Prescription drugs are considered safe for use only with medical supervision and can be dispensed only with a prescription from a licensed professional with governmental privileges to prescribe. Examples of such professionals are physicians, dentists, nurse practitioners, physician's assistants, or veterinarians. Nonprescription drugs are considered safe for use without a prescription.

These drugs are said to be available "over-the-counter," because you can walk up and buy them without a prescription. Examples of such medicines include aspirin and some cold and allergy medicines.

In the United States, the Food and Drug Administration (FDA) is the government agency that decides which drugs

Drug Names

All drugs have at least three names. These include a chemical name, a generic (nonproprietary or official) name, and a trade (proprietary or brand) name. The chemical name describes the atomic or molecular structure of the chemical itself. This name is usually too cumbersome for general use. So usually, a government body assigns a generic name to a drug. The generic names for drugs of a particular type (or class) usually have the same ending. For example, the names of all beta-blockers, which are used to treat such diseases as high blood pressure, end in "olol." The pharmaceutical company that manufactures or distributes the drug chooses a brand name. Patented drugs are usually sold under a brand name. Generic versions of brand-name drugs may be sold under the generic name. For example, the nonprescription painkiller ibuprofen is sold under many different brand names including Advil®, Motrin®, and Nuprin®.

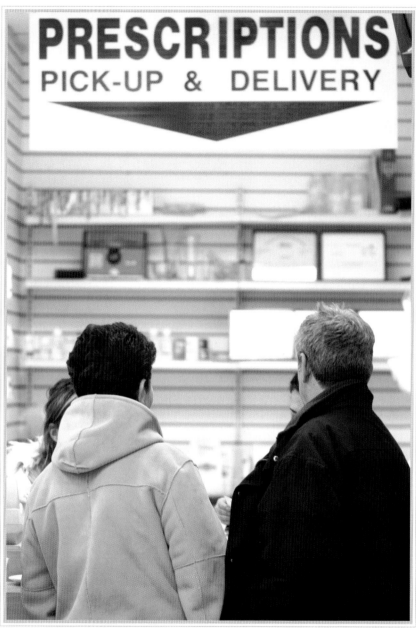

Prescription medicines can only be purchased with the pharmacist's help, while over-the-counter medications can simply be picked up off the drugstore shelves and purchased.

are legal to sell. It also decides if a drug should require a prescription or if it may be sold over-the-counter. This law does
not cover alternative medicines, such as vitamins, nutritional
supplements, and medicinal herbs; this means they have not
undergone the comprehensive testing required by the FDA.
Canada has an organization similar to the FDA, called the
Therapeutic Product Directorate (TPD). The TPD is a di-
vision of Health Canada, the Canadian government depart-
ment of health. The TPD regulates drugs, medical devices,
disinfectants, and sanitizers with disinfectant claims. Some
of the things the TPD monitors are quality, effectiveness, and
safety. Just as the FDA must approve new drugs in the United

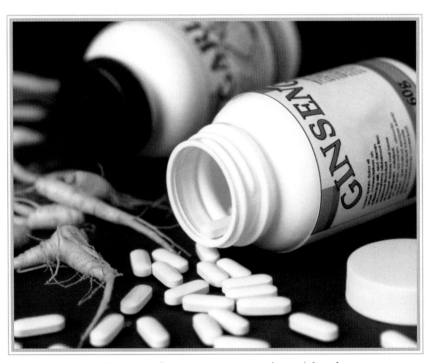

"Natural" remedies are not regulated by the FDA.

How Are Drugs Classified?

Generally, drugs are classified by the disorder or symptom they are used to treat. For example, drugs used to treat high blood pressure are called antihypertensives, and drugs used to treat depression are called antidepressants. Within each therapeutic group, drugs are categorized by classes. Some classes are based on how the drugs work in the body. For instance, selective serotonin reuptake inhibitors (SSRIs) are so named because they interfere with serotonin reuptake in the brain.

States, the TPD must approve new drugs in Canada before those drugs can enter the market.

How Drugs Are Developed

Many of the drugs we use today were discovered by experiments conducted on animals and humans. Now, many drugs are being designed with the specific disease in mind: once the abnormal biochemical and cellular changes caused by disease are identified, compounds that may specifically prevent or correct these abnormalities (by interacting with specific sites in the body) can be designed. If a new compound shows promise, its structure is usually changed several times to increase its ability to target the intended site (selectivity) and remain attached to the site (affinity). It may also be altered to

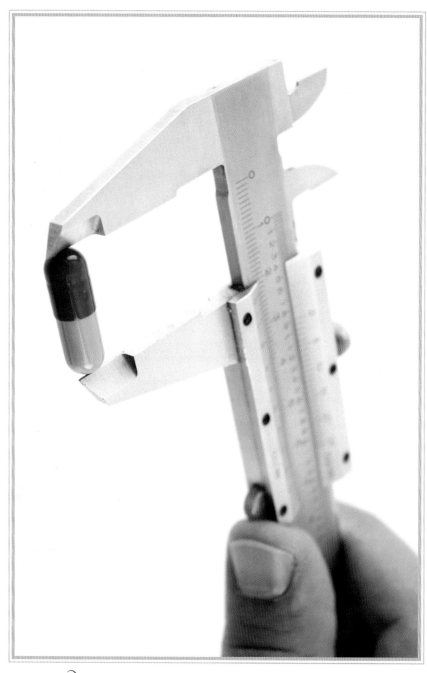

Standard dose—the exact amount of a medication needed—is determined during drug development.

optimize its strength (potency), effectiveness (efficacy), and safety. Other factors, such as how the body absorbs the compound and whether it is stable in body tissues and fluids, are also considered. These factors involve what the body does to the drug and what the drug does to the body.

A drug will usually be successful when it is highly selective for its target site, so that it has little or no effect on other body systems; that is, it has few side effects. The drug should also be very potent and effective, so that low doses can be used, even for diseases that are hard to treat. The drug should be effective when taken by mouth (for convenient administration), absorbed well from the digestive tract, and reasonably stable in body tissues and fluids, so that ideally, one dose a day is adequate.

During the course of drug development, standard or average doses are determined. However, all people respond to drugs differently. Many factors, including age, weight, genetics, and the presence of other illnesses or medications, affect drug response. These factors must be considered when doctors prescribe any medicine for a particular patient.

The main goals of drug development are effectiveness and safety. Since drugs can harm as well as help, safety is relative. The difference between the usual effective dose and the dose that produces severe or life-threatening side effects is called the margin of safety. The larger the margin of safety, the safer the drug in clinical practice. If a drug's usual effective dose is toxic, doctors do not use the drug unless the situation is serious and there is no better alternative. The most beneficial

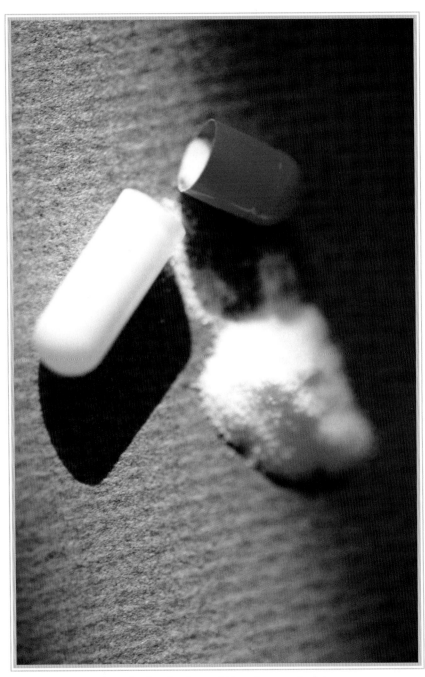

*A placebo looks just like the real thing—
but it contains no active ingredients.*

drugs are effective and safe. Penicillin is an example of such a drug. Except for people who are allergic to it, penicillin is almost completely nontoxic, even in large doses. On the other hand, barbiturates, which were once commonly prescribed to help people sleep, can interfere with breathing, lower blood pressure, and even cause death if they are taken in excess.

Designing effective drugs with a wide margin of safety and few side effects is sometimes very difficult. As a result, some drugs must be used even though they have a very narrow margin of safety. For example, warfarin (Coumadin®), which is taken to prevent blood clotting, can cause dangerous bleeding, but it is used when the need to thin the blood is so great that the risk must be accepted. People who take this drug need frequent testing to see whether the drug is causing the blood to clot too much, too little, or the desired amount.

When testing to see if a drug is effective, scientists sometimes use a placebo. A placebo is made to look exactly like a real drug but is made of an inactive substance such as a starch or sugar. Sometimes people improve on their own, without treatment. If a change, either positive or negative, occurs after a placebo is taken, this may be because the person *thought* she was receiving treatment, and the power of her belief helped her to get well. This is called the "placebo effect."

Some people seem more susceptible to the placebo effect than others. People who have a positive opinion of drugs, doctors, nurses, and hospitals are more likely to respond favorably to placebos than are people who have a negative opinion. So when a new drug is being developed, researchers conduct studies to compare the effect of the drug with that of a placebo, because a drug that doesn't work can still have a placebo effect. The true effectiveness of the drug must be distinguished from a placebo effect. Half the study's participants are given the drug, and half are given an identical-looking placebo. When neither the participants nor the doctors know who received the drug and who received the placebo it is called a "double-blind" study.

When a study is completed, all changes observed in participants taking the actual drug are compared with those in participants taking the placebo. The drug must perform much better than the placebo to justify its use. In some studies, as many as half of the participants taking the placebo improve (an example of the placebo effect), making it difficult to determine the effectiveness of the drug being tested.

The Stages of Drug Development

For every 10,000 compounds that are screened in the laboratory, approximately 1,000 of them make it to the preclinical stage. Preclinical testing usually consists of laboratory tests on animals. Of those, perhaps ten reach Phase I clinical studies, five advance into Phase III clinical studies, and in the end, out of the original 10,000 compounds, perhaps only one is ultimately ever approved for marketing. Developing a new drug is a long, expensive process that may take from ten to twelve years or more. Typically, the process involves several steps including drug discovery, preclinical testing, clinical testing, and application for FDA approval for marketing.

After preclinical testing in animals, human clinical trials are typically conducted in three phases:

- Phase I studies are designed to determine the safety of a new drug. These studies are small, typically involving fewer than forty patients, and are used to identify side effects and the maximum tolerated dose of the drug. Further trials and development cannot take place unless Phase I trials show the drug to be safe when administered to humans.

- Phase II studies are designed to confirm the safety of the drug, determine whether the drug may be effective in humans, and gather data for the larger Phase III clinical trials. Phase II studies are larger than Phase I studies, typically enrolling up to one hundred patients.

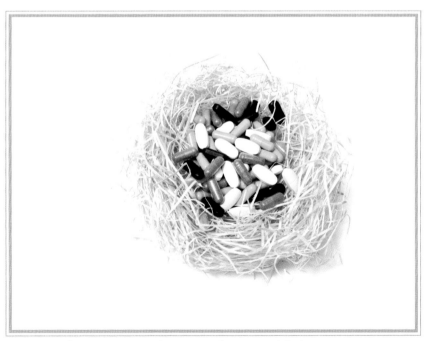

"Hatching" a new drug is a long and laborious process.

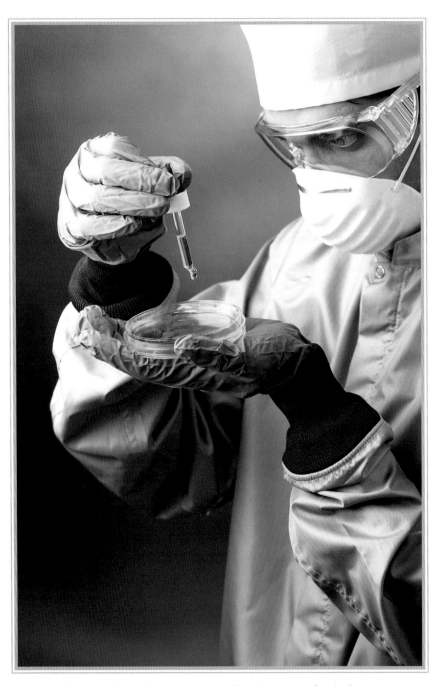

Preclinical trials are typically done in the laboratory; after that, testing takes place with real human beings.

- Phase III studies are designed to provide convincing evidence of the safety and effectiveness of the drug by comparing it against another standard medication or treatment. Phase III studies are usually large, enrolling hundreds or even thousands of patients, sometimes for long periods of time. In most cases, they are controlled and double-blinded to provide the most convincing evidence for the safety and efficacy of the drug.

Phase I and II studies can be completed in as little as one or two years, while Phase III studies typically require three years or more before all the results have been analyzed.

In the United States, once all the clinical data is collected and analyzed and there is convincing evidence of the safety and efficacy of the drug, a new drug application (NDA) is filed and reviewed by the FDA. After review, the FDA may approve the drug for sale, request additional clinical information, or deny approval. After drugs have been approved for marketing, Phase IV studies may be performed to explore new indications, long-term safety, or drug interactions.

When a company develops a new drug, it can be granted a *patent* for the drug itself, for the way the drug is made, for the way the drug is to be used, and even for the method of delivering and releasing the drug into the bloodstream. Usually a company owns several patents for each drug. Patents grant the company exclusive rights to a drug for twenty years. Often, by the time a drug is discovered (when a patent is obtained) and when it is approved for use, only about half the patent time is left to exclusively market a new drug. Once a patent has expired, other companies may produce and sell a

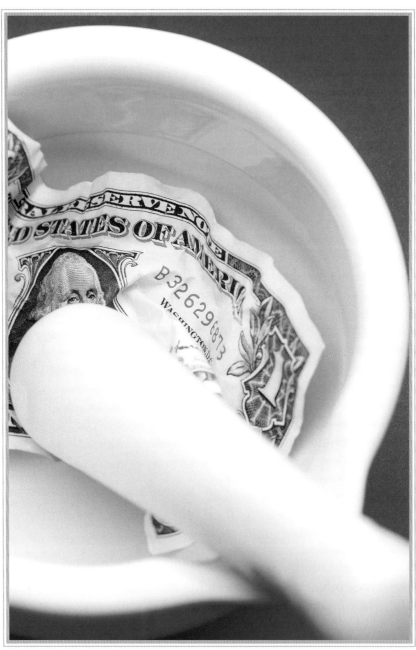

Drug development is a costly process—that ultimately reaps enormous economic payoffs for pharmaceutical companies.

generic version of the drug, typically at a much lower price than the original trade-name drug.

Drug companies devote considerable time, energy, and dollars to developing new medications—and depression is currently one of the "big" diseases on which pharmaceuticals are focusing their efforts. In today's world, depression is more often diagnosed than it was in previous generations—but there are also better weapons to combat this disease.

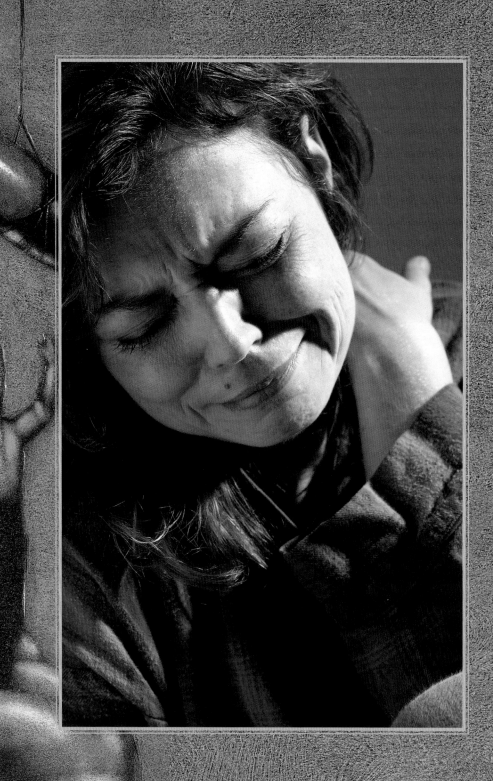

Chapter 5

Better Weapons in the War on Depression

S andra was losing hope. Her friend Georgia was back in the hospital again; her depression had gotten so bad the doctors were afraid she might hurt herself. As Sandra stood in the hospital corridor, with white-coated doctors hurrying past, she wondered why all these bright people with all their years of schooling and experience had not yet found anything that could help her best friend get her life back.

Sandra was there to support Georgia's mom and dad when they went to meet with the doctors who were in charge of Georgia's care. As this was Georgia's third hospitalization, the atmosphere in the small conference room was grim. Georgia's mother cried as the doctors described the treatment options available for Georgia, the drugs they hadn't already tried, even the possibility of **shock therapy**. A young resident was a part of the conference as well.

As Georgia's mom began to cry harder, the resident leaned across the coffee table and held the crying woman's hand in his own. "You shouldn't give up hope," he said. "There are still several things that we haven't tried, and there are always new treatments being developed. Ten years from now, Georgia may be enjoying a rich and successful life thanks to a treatment that is still in clinical trials today. What is important now is that your daughter is getting help. As long as she stays in treatment, there is always hope."

When Sandra left the hospital that afternoon, she thought about the young doctor's optimism. When she reached her home, she went straight to her computer and got online. She couldn't wait to see what new treatments scientists were working on to help her friend.

Serotonin Reuptake

To visualize the process of serotonin reuptake, imagine a vacuum cleaner that sucks the serotonin back into the cell. SSRIs block the vacuum, the way your family's vacuum cleaner might get blocked if you were to suck up a sock or some other large object. When the vacuum is clogged, nothing else can get sucked up. When this happens in the cell, it leaves the serotonin in the synapse to be used again, which means the amount of available serotonin in the synapse is increased.

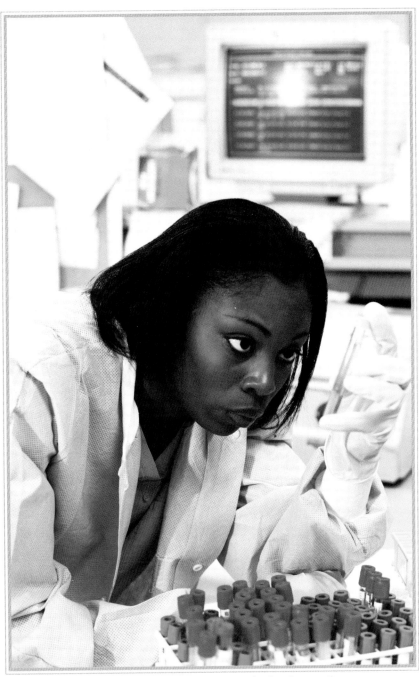

*Scientists are constantly looking for
better treatments for depression.*

Most currently available antidepressants can be classified as belonging to one of several major classes: monoamine oxidase inhibitors (MAOIs), tricyclic antidepressants (TCAs), or selective serotonin reuptake inhibitors (SSRIs). The newest classes of antidepressants currently available to patients are norepinephrine reuptake inhibitors (NRIs), and combined serotonin/norepinephrine reuptake inhibitors (SNRIs).

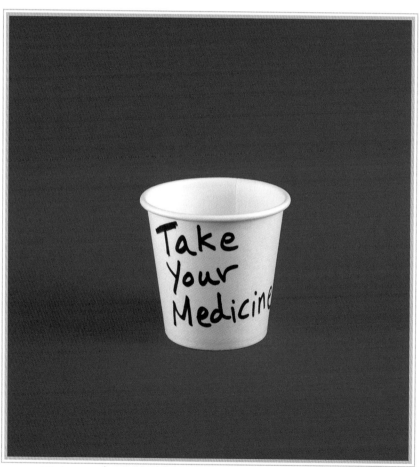

SSRIs are the most frequently prescribed treatment for depression in the United States.

Reuptake Inhibitors

SSRIs have become the dominant treatment for depression in the United States, mostly because they cause fewer side effects than other drugs that are available. However, recent evidence indicates that less selective compounds may work better than the SSRIs. Currently available "dual reuptake inhibitors," SNRIs, include milnacipran, venlafaxine, and duloxetine. Venlafaxine, sold under the brand name Effexor XR®, was the first commercially available antidepressant in this new drug class.

Duloxetine (Cymbalta®) also acts on both serotonin and norepinephrine. This drug was granted FDA approval in the summer of 2004 for treatment of major depressive disorder (as well as ***diabetic peripheral neuropathic pain***) and is one of the newest antidepressants on the market. Side effects are generally mild and include dry mouth, nausea, and sleepiness. Milnacipran (Ixel®) is a similar drug that is not yet FDA approved for sale in the United States. It is specifically being researched for helping people with ***fibromyalgia*** as well as the treatment of depression.

Nefazodone (Serzone®) is another SNRI. Nefazodone is more rapidly effective and has fewer upsetting side effects (such as sexual dysfunction and sleep disorders) than SSRIs. Unfortunately, nefazodone has recently been linked with increased risk of liver failure. Patients should consult their physician concerning the risks and benefits of taking this medication. The drug was withdrawn from the Canadian market in 2003 due the risk of liver failure, but it is still available in the United States (although it is rarely used).

Two newer SNRIs, reboxetine and atomoxetine, may soon be available. These drugs make norepinephrine more available without the same side effects or dangers as the older TCAs. So far, reboxetine, which is not yet on the American market, has shown effectiveness in treating depression and anxiety disorders, and is speculated to be effective in treating *attention deficit disorder* as well. Atomoxetine is marketed in the United States as Strattera® and has shown to alleviate attention deficit disorder. Research is currently under way to see if Strattera will prove effective for depression as well.

NaSSA

Mirtazapine (Remeron®) is a relatively new antidepressant that is referred to as a NaSSA, or noradrenergic and specific serotonergic antidepressant. Mirtazapine may indirectly enhance the effects of both serotonin and norepinephrine. Compared to some common SSRIs, studies indicate that it works more rapidly and is effective against anxiety in patients with both anxiety and depression. It also improves sleep. Patients are able to safely switch directly from an SSRI to mirtazapine without having to go through a withdrawal period. It may, however, elevate cholesterol and *triglyceride levels* slightly. It can also cause blurred vision and may cause weight gain.

MAOIs

MAOIs block the enzyme monoamine oxidase, which breaks down many of the neurotransmitters that are important for well-being. Commonly prescribed MAOIs include phenelzine (Nardil®), isocarboxazid (Marplan®), and tranylcypromine

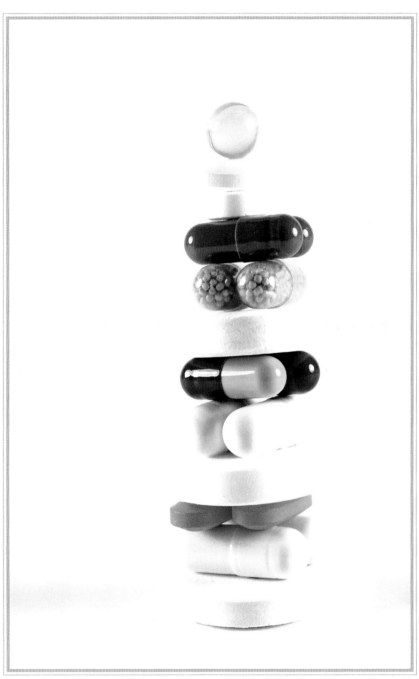

*There are many options to choose from in
today's world of antidepressants.*

(Parnate®). Because these agents can have very severe side effects, they are usually used only when other antidepressants prove ineffective.

However, new MAOIs are being developed, such as selegiline, to target only one form of the MAOI enzyme. Studies indicate these new drugs may be effective without the significant side effects of the older MAOIs. Recent studies have shown that selegiline delivered from a skin patch was effective and safe for patients with major depression and didn't cause any of the digestive upset caused by many antidepressants.

New Drugs Under Study

SP Inhibitors

Researchers are working hard to develop better, more effective treatments for depression all the time. One major new class of compounds under study for the treatment of depression is Substance P (SP) inhibitors, which are involved in pain and inflammation pathways and perhaps in the regulation of emotion. SP serves as a pain neurotransmitter, and it is involved in a variety of other functions, including breathing, circulation, salivation, and smooth muscle contraction in the digestive tract. SP blockers have also recently attracted interest as possible antidepressants.

Findings in recent preclinical studies have provided much of the drive to continue investigating the potential value of SP blockers in treating psychiatric disorders, particularly when these agents have not been effective for pain relief. When levels of SP are increased in animals, researchers have seen behavioral and cardiovascular effects resembling the stress response, the so-called "fight-or-flight response." Moreover, preclinical studies have shown a reduction of these behavioral and cardiovascular stress responses by interfering with SP receptors. A breakthrough study by Merck pharmaceuticals indicated that an SP receptor antagonist called MK-869 was more effective than a placebo, had no sexual side effects,

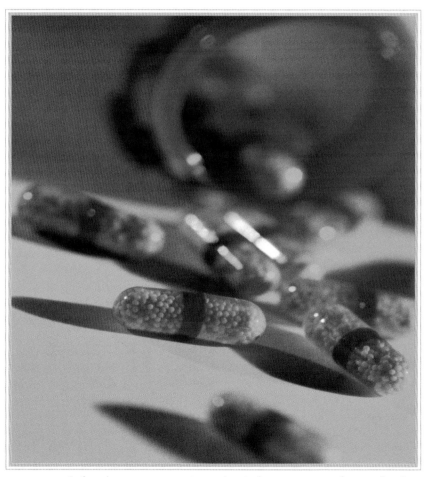

One of the dangers associated with MAOIs is the risk of overdose: taking too many pills at once can even be lethal.

and was as effective as a commonly prescribed antidepressant in patients with moderate to severe depression. A follow-up study was later unsuccessful, but another Merck SP targeted medication also proved to have a positive effect on major depression. MK-869 is still under active study for both depression and anxiety disorders.

FAAH Blockers

Anandamide is an important neurotransmitter since it affects mood, memory, pain, appetite, response to stress, and many other physiological processes. Scientists have identified the enzyme in the brain that **hydrolyzes** anandamide. It is called FAAH, an abbreviation for the fatty acid amide hydro-

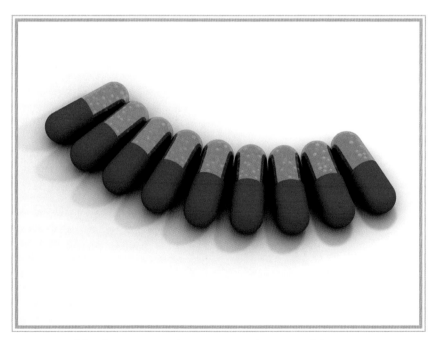

FAAH blockers may elevate people's mood by increasing the level of a particular neurotransmitter in the brain.

lase. Blocking the action of FAAH may help to increase anandamide levels, helping to elevate a person's mood. Two new FAAH blockers, SSR 101010 and SSR 411298, are currently being studied by the pharmaceutical company Sanofi-Aventis as a possible new class of antidepressants. FAAH is a controversial treatment option that is still being researched.

Mifepristone

Mifepristone (also known as RU-486, the same drug as the "morning-after pill" which is prescribed as an abortion measure, although it is prescribed in different doses for depression.) is a powerful glucocorticoid (GR II) receptor blocker. The basic idea behind this potential antidepressant is that mifepristone interferes with the action of GR II. Several recent studies have suggested that blocking the action of GR II may be a potential treatment strategy for major depression with psychotic features, as elevated cortisol levels are particularly common in this kind of depression. A small, double-blind, placebo-controlled study was recently completed with five subjects, three men and two women. In this study, patients received four days of placebo followed by 600 milligrams mifepristone, or vice versa.

Outcome measures were standard tests used to rate depression. During the mifepristone administration, there was a 34 percent decrease in the score that rates the severity of a patient's depression on one test. Scores on the same rating scale later increased by 1 percent during the placebo phase. Using another test, doctors found that scores indicating depression declined by 26 percent during the mifepristone phase, while they went down by only 6 percent during the placebo phase. This study clearly suggested that disruption of GR II function could result in the improvement of psychiatric symptoms.

A larger multisite study has also been completed in which patients with psychotic major depression received 50 milligrams, 600 milligrams, or 1,200 milligrams per day of mifepristone for 7 days; this study was not double-blinded, but it demonstrated that mifepristone caused a rapid reduction in symptoms, with a greater response to treatment with increased dosage. These studies are very promising as they suggest the possibility of a rapid and effective treatment for psychotic depression; more will be understood about this drug following the results of current Phase II and Phase III clinical trials.

What Makes These New Drugs Better?

Different kinds of drugs create different side effects and problems. Currently available drugs often bring relief from symptoms only to cause problematic side effects.

The class of drugs known as MAOIs, for example, can be toxic at the wrong dose. Patients taking these medications have to be carefully monitored by a psychiatrist. MAOIs can also have some very unpleasant side effects. These include weight gain, fluid retention, sleeplessness, headaches, fatigue, stomach problems, and anxiety. Some patients refuse to take these drugs because they would rather be depressed than deal with the physical effects of the medicine. MAOIs can also interact with certain foods, resulting in a restricted diet for the patient.

Meanwhile, the TCAs are easier to dose than MAOIs and have fewer side effects, but they can still cause very real problems for many of the people taking them. They often affect glandular function throughout the body, so dry eyes, dry mouth, and constipation are all common complaints from people taking these drugs. Drowsiness is another major side effect, and many patients complain of feeling "drugged" while taking these medicines. Nausea and weight gain are also common side effects; less common is a sharp drop in blood pressure.

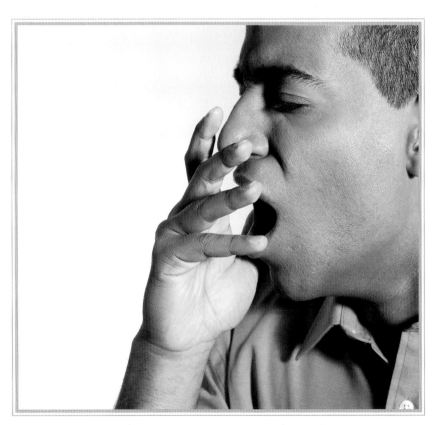

Antidepressants can cause drowsiness.

These drugs can often take a month to work, causing a great hardship for people struggling with depression. Before they had their illness to deal with, which was bad enough. Now, for the first four weeks of treatment, they are coping with depression plus a host of unpleasant physical side effects. For this reason, scientists are working hard to design newer, quicker-acting drugs.

Although SSRIs have far fewer side effects than their predecessors, they still can produce side effects that cause some people to discontinue treatment. Side effects include nausea, diarrhea, headache, and anxiety. Other people complain of fatigue, and SSRIs can cause minor sleep disruptions. Weight gain can also be an issue after the first six months.

Again, researchers are always on the lookout for drugs that can produce the same effect with fewer unwanted side effects. Since many side effects involve the digestive system, researchers are investigating new methods of delivery that bypass the digestive tract, such as delivering medication through a skin patch. The patch may be available on the U.S. market within the next couple of years.

New Nondrug Treatments

New alternatives to medication are also emerging as research continues. **Vagus nerve** stimulation, or VNS therapy, has helped thousands of people whose **epilepsy** did not respond to medication, and the FDA has recently approved it for treating depression as well. An electronic device is surgically implanted in the patient's chest, and then a wire sends an electrical charge through the vagus nerve. It is thought that this

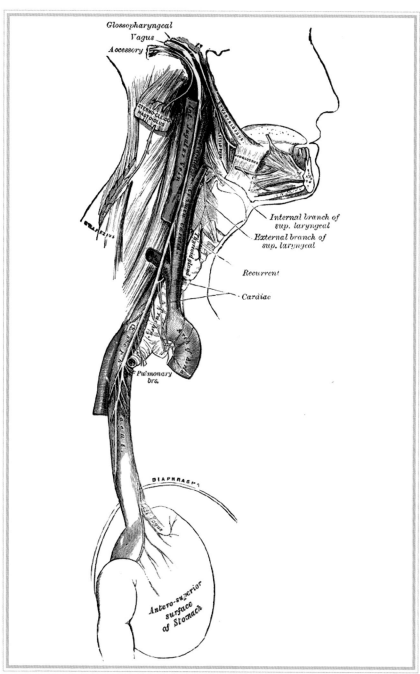

The vagus nerve (shown here in yellow)
travels up through the body to the brain.

increases the brain's production of important brain chemicals related to depression. After the patient recovers from surgery, the stimulation is painless, and the most common side effect associated with the treatment is a slight hoarseness that fades over time.

Positron-emission tomography (PET) studies show changes in critical brain areas during VNS treatment. A study performed on sixty patients with treatment-resistant major depression also showed significant improvement after VNS treatment. Better response rates were seen in patients with low to moderate antidepressant resistance than in extremely treatment-resistant patients. Long-term studies are still nec-

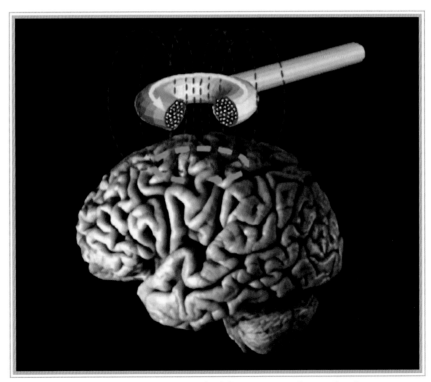

TMS uses a magnetic field to stimulate the brain.

essary to determine what role, if any, VNS will play in treatment-resistant depression.

Another alternative approach to the treatment of depression is the use of transcranial magnetic stimulation (TMS). In TMS, an electromagnetic coil is placed on the scalp, through which a high-intensity current is rapidly turned on and off, resulting in a magnetic field. The coil is held onto the scalp (although no actual contact is necessary), and the magnetic field passes through the skull and into the brain. Small induced currents can then make brain areas below the coil more or less active, depending on the settings used.

In practice, TMS can influence many brain functions, including movement, visual perception, memory, reaction time, speech, and mood. The effects produced are genuine but temporary, lasting only a short time after actual stimulation has stopped. Since it is believed that some mental disorders are the result of over- or underactive nerve cells, successful treatment could be achieved by modifying these cells' behavior. The range of effects produced by TMS gives scientists hope of its potential to work in this way.

Risks and Benefits of Experimental Treatments

Because there are still many people struggling with treatment-resistant depression, participating in a clinical trial for an experimental treatment can have great appeal. Participants in clinical trials are anxious to have access to cutting-edge treatments not currently available elsewhere. However, these treatments are indeed experimental and can have risks. For individuals considering an experimental drug, there are several factors to consider before making a final decision.

All clinical trials in the United States are reviewed and monitored by an Institutional Review Board (IRB). This board consists of a group of independent physicians, **statisticians**, community **advocates**, and others who work to ensure that the clinical trials are as low risk to the patients as possible. But the purpose of a clinical trial is to investigate the risks of the particular treatment. As a result, the physicians involved may not yet know any potential risks or side effects.

There is also no guarantee a patient will receive the investigational drug. Most clinical trials use a control group on which to base the treatment effects. This means that when someone decides to participate in a clinical trial and is accepted, he may or may not receive the treatment being studied. Participants must accept the possibility that they could receive placebos.

On the other hand, there are also a lot of benefits to participating in a clinical trial. Most clinical trials are held in top-notch facilities with doctors who are experts in their fields. Because of the amount of money that the pharmaceutical industry pours into research and development, drug companies are very cautious in choosing the physicians who will participate in the final clinical trial. By participating in the trial, patients gain access to not only the new treatments before they are available, but they also are under the care of a very qualified physician.

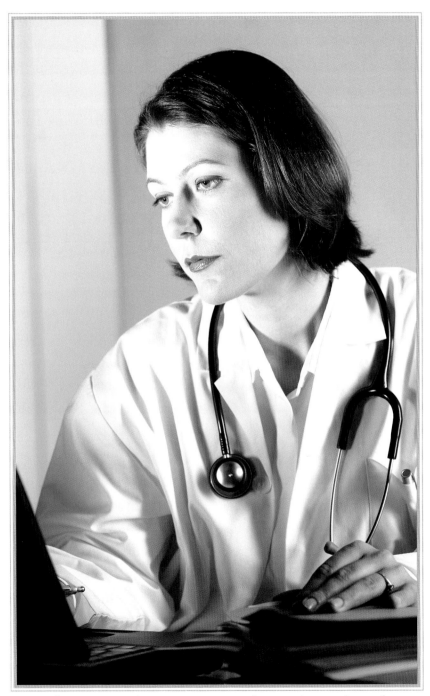

Physicians play important roles in clinical trials.

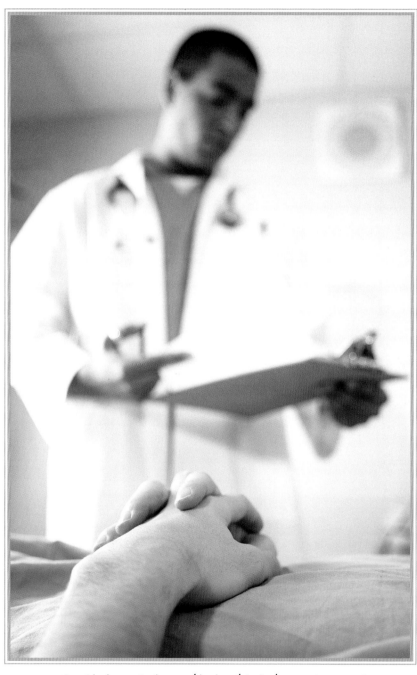

*Participants in a clinical trial must report
regularly to the study physician.*

Getting accepted into a clinical trial is often not easy. All clinical trials are based on a series of "rules" that determine how the clinical trial will be held and what type of patient can participate. These can include criteria such as:

- The patient must be a certain age.

- The patient must be in relative good health.

- The patient must not be in another clinical trial.

- The patient must have the specific type and severity of illness that the drug is intended to treat.

Many times, a clinical trial requires participants to be more active than usual in their treatment. Some of the requirements include routine checkups and visits with the study physician, often up to two years after receiving the new treatment. Participants may be required to report for special tests. There are also financial considerations, since many health insurance providers will not cover an experimental treatment, although often patients in these trials are treated for free.

The process by which new antidepressants are created, tested, and marketed is lengthy and expensive. However, the results for people affected by this debilitating illness make worthwhile the tremendous level of effort and expense. As scientists begin to understand more fully the causes of the illness, the future for people struggling with depression looks brighter now than it has for many decades. This increased understanding has opened up a whole new range of treatments for people with depression.

Further Reading

Dunbar, Katherine. *Antidepressants.* Farmington Hills, Mich.: Thomson Gale, 2005.

Ford, Jean. *Antidepressants and the Critics: Cure-Alls or Unnatural Poisons?* Broomall, Pa.: Mason Crest, 2007.

Esherick, Joan. *The FDA and Psychiatric Drugs: How a Drug Is Approved.* Broomall, Pa.: Mason Crest, 2004.

Hunter, David. *Antidepressants and the Pharmaceutical Companies: Corporate Responsibilities.* Broomall, Pa.: Mason Crest, 2007.

Koplewicz, Harold S. *More than Moody: Recognizing and Treating Adolescent Depression.* New York: Penguin, 2003.

McIntosh, Kenneth. *The History of Depression: The Mind–Body Connection.* Broomall, Pa.: Mason Crest, 2007.

Russell, Craig. *Antidepressants and Their Side Effects: Managing the Risks.* Broomall, Pa.: Mason Crest, 2007.

Walker, Maryalice. *The Development of Antidepressants: The Chemistry of Depression.* Broomall, Pa.: Mason Crest, 2007.

Wurtzel, Elizabeth. *Prozac Nation: Young and Depressed in America.* New York: Penguin, 2002.

For More Information

Association of Clinical Research Professionals
500 Montgomery Street, Suite 800
Alexandria, VA 22314
Tel.: (703) 254-8100
Fax: (703) 254-8101
www.acrpnet.org

Depression and Bipolar Support Alliance
730 N. Franklin Street, Suite 501
Chicago, IL 60610-7224
Tel.: (800) 826-3632
Fax: (312) 642-7243
www.dbsalliance.org

National Alliance for the Mentally Ill
Colonial Place Three
2107 Wilson Blvd., Suite 300
Arlington, VA 22201-3042
Tel.: (703) 524-7600
Fax: (703) 524-9094
www.nami.org

National Institute of Mental Health (NIMH)
Public Information and Communications Branch
6001 Executive Boulevard, Room 8184, MSC 9663
Bethesda, MD 20892-9663
Tel.: (866) 615-6464
Fax: (301) 443-4279
www.nimh.nih.gov

National Mental Health Association
2001 N. Beauregard Street, 12th Floor
Alexandria, VA 22311
Tel.: (703) 684-7722
Fax: (703) 684-5968
www.nmha.org

The New Drug Approval Process
www.fda.gov/cder/handbook/develop.htm

Teens' Health: Depression
kidshealth.org/teen/your_mind/mental_health/depression.
html

Publisher's note:
The Web sites listed on these pages were active at the time of publication. The publisher is not responsible for Web sites that have changed their addresses or discontinued operation since the date of publication. The publisher will review and update the Web-site list upon each reprint.

Glossary

advocates: People who support or speak in favor of something.

amygdala: An almond-shaped mass, one in each hemisphere of the brain, associated with feelings of fear and aggression and important for visual learning and memory.

attention deficit disorder: A condition characterized by hyperactivity, inability to concentrate, and impulsive or inappropriate behavior.

autonomic responses: The body's involuntary activities, such as heartbeat and digestion.

bipolar disorder: A psychiatric disorder characterized by extreme emotional highs and lows; sometimes called manic-depressive disorder.

cerebrospinal: Involving the brain and spinal cord.

chronic: Something that is long-lasting or recurs frequently.

clinical depression: An observable state of sadness or melancolia that disrupts an individual's daily activities.

diabetic peripheral neuropathic pain: Discomfort caused by an abnormality in the nervous system of someone with diabetes.

epilepsy: A medical disorder involving periods of abnormal electrical discharges in the brain and characterized by periodic sudden loss or impairment of consciousness, often accompanied by convulsions.

estrogen: The hormones produced in the ovaries that stimulate the menstrual cycle and the development of secondary sexual characteristics.

fibromyalgia: A disorder causing aching muscles, sleep disorders, and fatigue.

hormones: Chemical substances produced in the body that have a regulatory or stimulatory effect.

hydrolyzes: Makes a substance undergo a chemical reaction in which a compound reacts with water, causing decomposition and the production of two or more other compounds.

limbic system: An interconnected system of brain nuclei associated with basic needs and emotions.

mania: A period of extreme emotional highs and physical activity.

neurons: Cells that transmit nerve impulses.

neurotransmitters: Chemicals that carry messages between nerve cells.

patent: An exclusive right granted by the government to an inventor to make or sell an invention.

postmenopausal: Occurring after menopause, the time when a woman stops menstruating.

postpartum: Occurring in or relating to the period immediately following childbirth.

sensitized: Induced a heightened reaction to a particular substance.

shock therapy: A method of treating patients with psychiatric disorders involving the passing of an electric current through the brain.

spontaneously: Occurring naturally, without apparent external influence.

statisticians: People who compile and work with the collection, analysis, interpretation, and presentation of masses of numerical data.

triglyceride levels: The amount of the chemical compound formed from a molecule of the alcohol glycerol and three molecules of fatty acids in the body.

vagus nerve: Either of the tenth pair of nerves within the skull that carries sensory and motor neurons, serving the heart, lungs, stomach, intestines, and other organs.

vulnerability: The inability to resist illness or debility.

Bibliography

American Academy of Family Physicians. http://www.aafp.org.

Brown, Richard, Teodoro Bottiglieri, and Carol Colman. *Stop Depression Now*. New York: Berkley Books, 2000.

Depression and the Pharmaceutical Industry. http://www.abpi.org.uk.

Donovan, Charles E. *Out of the Black Hole*. St. Louis, Mo.: Wellness Publishers, 2005.

McMan's Depression and Bipolar Web. http://www.mcmanweb.com.

National Depressive and Manic-Depressive Association. http://www.ndmda.org.

Recovery Inc. http://www.recovery-inc.com.

Web MD. http://www.webmd.com.

Index

Picture Credits

Benjamin Stewart: pp. 17, 37

Comstock Images: p. 81

Gray's Anatomy: pp. 44, 87

iStockphotos: pp. 14, 24, 38, 48, 79

    Amanda Rohde: p. 67

    Andrew Wood: p. 52

    Andy Green: p. 26

    Chris Hellyar: p. 62

    Dawn Johnston: p. 43

    Edyta Pawlowska: p. 47

    Jonathan Coombs: p. 76

    Joseph Jean Rolland Dubé: p. 34

    Lev Mel: p. 82

    Maartje van Caspel: pp. 30, 33

    Maciej Laska: p. 8

    Natalia Bratslavsky: p. 59

    Thomas Reekie: p. 11

Jupiter Images: pp. 18, 20, 41, 50, 54, 56, 60, 64, 68, 70, 72, 75, 85, 91, 92

Malinda Miller: p. 29

National Institute of Health: p. 88

Biographies

Author

Heather Docalavich has written a number of books for young people on a wide variety of topics. She resides in Hilton Head Island, South Carolina, with her four children.

Consultant

Andrew M. Kleiman, M.D., received a Bachelor of Arts degree in philosophy from the University of Michigan, and earned his medical degree from Tulane University School of Medicine. Dr. Kleiman completed his internship, residency in psychiatry, and fellowship in forensic psychiatry at New York University and Bellevue Hospital. He is currently in private practice in Manhattan, specializing in psychopharmacology, psychotherapy, and forensic psychiatry. He also teaches clinical psychology at the New York University School of Medicine.